The Pregnancy Weight Book™

Your guide to a happy, healthy pregnancy

by

Adriana Martin

Fitness Guru, Weight Loss Coach and Mom

Disclaimer

The facts and opinions are presented for informational purposes only and are not a substitute for professional medical advice. Any action taken in response to the information provided in this book is at the reader's discretion.

You should consult a physician in all matters relating to your health prior to starting a health and wellness regimen, and particularly with respect to any symptoms that may require diagnosis or medical attention.

Table of Contents

Introduction

Congratulations! You're pregnant. This is a joyful time in your life and there's no time like the present to discover all the things you can do to ensure a happy, healthy pregnancy.

I'm honored that you've chosen me as your guide to a safe, simple approach to diet and exercise. Being your teacher is a responsibility I take seriously. And I've packed tons of useful information for you in the pages to come.

But this isn't a dry, heavy, academic book. Along with do's and don'ts, whys and why nots, I've done my best to include some wit and humor to keep you motivated and inspired.

Are you ready to stay in great shape during the next nine months? You've come to the right place. **The Pregnancy Weight Book** ™ reveals the secrets for prenatal fitness, healthy eating options, and tips for ways YOU can enjoy a vigorous and beautiful pregnancy.

No pressure! (And no "tests" either.) There is no right or wrong way to approach this learning experience. By that I mean that you don't have to read this book in order! Just find the topic that you're more interested in and jump right in. I guarantee you'll find what you're looking for here!

My hope is that this book will be the beginning of a long and fruitful relationship. And from now on I want you to think of me as your pre- and post-natal fitness coach!

Your questions, comments and feedback are important to me and I want to hear from you!

So if you need more information, additional details, or just want to say "Hi, Adriana," please visit me at www.AdrianaMartin.com

What You'll Learn

I've broken the book down in three categories... the foundational 'pillars' for experiencing a safe, healthy, pregnancy:

About Fitness	About Food	About You

- In the **About Fitness** section, you'll get answers to your fitness questions and learn a simple, but effective pre-natal workout that will keep you fit and strong before, during, and after your 'blessed event'
- In the **About Food** section, you'll get 'the skinny' on pre-natal nutrition so you know exactly what to do to gain the appropriate, recommended amount of extra pounds...while avoiding the unhealthy excess weight gain
- In the **About YOU** section, you'll learn powerful strategies that will allow you to enjoy and celebrate a peaceful, healthy, and in-shape pregnancy.

Staying in good shape during pregnancy is easier than you think! You only need three things to accomplish your goals:

- **A Willingness to Learn** – You've demonstrated that you have that when you ordered this book

- **A Plan** – I'll provide that in the following chapters

- **Commitment** – Staying healthy isn't hard, but it does require regular effort on your part

The Pregnancy Weight Book ™ includes your <u>pre-natal workout</u> as well as your <u>meal suggestion guide</u> and the <u>keys to staying in emotional harmony</u>. Working on these three components during the following nine months will help you stay in top shape both physically and emotionally.

Every Step of Your Journey Should Be Joyous

It's natural to be impatient when you're pregnant. After all, you're waiting for the birth of your beautiful son or daughter. But don't get ahead of yourself. In the months leading up to the arrival of your little one, it's important to focus on <u>enjoying the journey one day at a time</u>.

Discover the beauty of carrying a child inside of you. Marvel at the changes you feel. And make sure your body stays strong by working out every day and eating nutritiously so your baby has the best quality nutrients to develop healthfully.

But hold on for a moment. There's one important point you need to understand before we go one step further together...

Before You Begin

If ever there were a time to follow the 'better safe than sorry' rule, it's now! I can't stress this enough: you should **ALWAYS consult your doctor before starting an exercise program.** This is true even if you're not pregnant. However, you *are* pregnant, and it's especially vital that you have the input and support of your healthcare professional.

Be prepared, because I'm going to mention this point plenty of times throughout the program. Your doctor knows you and is familiar with your health history, and can raise a red flag if anything you are contemplating may be counter-indicated (a $10-word for 'not a good idea.')

I recommend that you show your doctor **The Pregnancy Weight Book™** and get his/her feedback on it! I'm sure he'll congratulate you for taking this valuable step.

Okay, now that's out of the way, the joyous work of finding health and balance can begin. Let's get started. Nine months goes by very quickly and you don't want to waste a moment.

ABOUT FITNESS

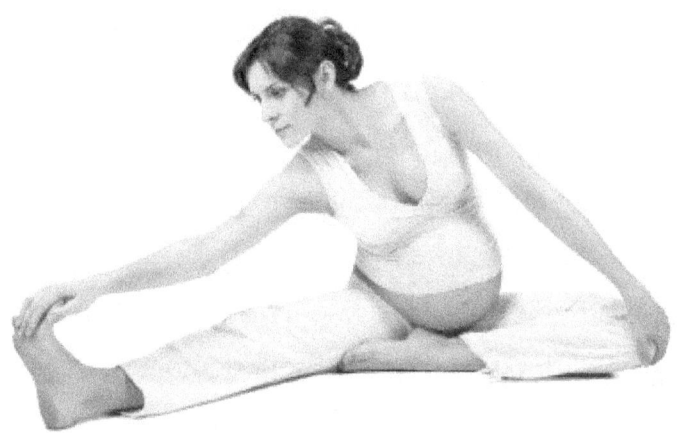

Pregnancy is NOT the time to get in shape. However, it IS the time to <u>stay in the best shape possible</u>. 'About Fitness' is your complete guide on how to safely and effectively exercise and stay fit during pregnancy.

What Are the Fitness/Exercise Guidelines I Need to Follow?

The rule of thumb when it comes to exercising during pregnancy is to always consult your doctor before starting. (I told you I was going to repeat this point). Your healthcare provider knows your body and baby's development better than I do. That's why I really must insist that you get his/her OK before you start this program.

Doctors' Recommendations

Once you get medical clearance, you've got the green light to get started. But you should also continue to monitor yourself and your body's response to **The Pregnancy Weight Book™** throughout your pregnancy.

According to the guidelines of The American Congress of Obstetricians and Gynecologists, you should stop exercising and call your doctor immediately if you experience any the following symptoms:

- Vaginal Bleeding
- Trouble Breathing
- Dizziness
- Severe Headache
- Chest Pain

- Muscle Weakness
- Preterm Labor
- Decreased Fetal Movement
- Amniotic Fluid Leakage
- Unusual Pain
- Uterine Contractions

9 Good Sense Safety Tips

Watching out for negative responses to exercise is the first and most important step. But here are some other guidelines that will help keep you safe and comfy during the process of staying fit:

1. **Always Listen to Your Body.** Your body knows best! So if you're feeling too tired or something just doesn't feel right, don't ignore the signals. It's best to stop, take a break, and get back on track later or the following day. And keep in mind: sometimes the best activity is no activity at all. Rest isn't just OK, it's part of the total picture of health.

2. **Avoid Laying On Your Back After the First Trimester** - As your uterus gets heavier it will press on the vein that returns blood from the lower body to your heart. Therefore, lying on your back for a long period of time could interfere with your baby's development. Not

to mention that your growing belly will press against the lungs making it hard for you to breathe.

3. **Wear Comfortable Shoes** – Your feet will have to support a lot of extra weight as your baby grows. Therefore it is important to find good support. Wearing good quality shoes that help distribute your weight evenly through the entire foot will avoid placing too much stress on your joints and back. (Save your spike-y Jimmy Choos and Manolo Blanicks for after the baby is born.)

4. **Put on a Good Bra** - Your breasts are preparing for lactation and you've undoubtedly noticed that they've grown beyond their 'normal' size. That's why it's important (and more comfortable) to wear the right support while exercising. This will help prevent your breasts from sagging and stretching and will also assist your back in supporting the extra weight.

5. **Dress Appropriately** – Your core temperature is higher than normal when you're pregnant. Therefore choosing light, loose clothing is important during this period as a way to stop your body from overheating. If you're exercising during the winter when lightweight clothing is inappropriate, just wear lots of layers so that you can peel them off as your body warms up.

6. **Drink Up** - Exercise saps a lot of water from your changing body; up to a quart during a vigorous workout. Since muscle movement depends on how hydrated you are, it's important that you stay hydrated in order to give your muscles what they need to bend, stretch, and workout. (For more info on the importance of water during pregnancy go to the About Food section of this program.)

7. **Warm Up** - Warming up before exercising builds your heart rate up gradually which, in turn, prepares your blood vessels to supply more blood and oxygen to the body. The right warm up can also prepare joints and muscles for bigger and more strenuous movements and that will enable you to get a better workout. Unfortunately, pregnant women who fail to warm up are more likely to experience faster fatigue and increase the risk for back pain and injury...so don't skip this important step.

8. **Cool Down** - Cooling down after working out is important for elite athletes, weekend warriors, and pregnant women. A cool down period allows you to decrease your heart rate and return your body's temperature to normal. During exercise your heart

pumps a lot faster, therefore distributing blood at a quicker pace. Since that blood has to return back into the heart your body assists it by muscular contraction and using the venous system. If you're exercising and stop suddenly your heart will continue to pump fast, but not receive the same amount of blood back which may cause you to feel dizzy.

9. **Stretch** - The best time to stretch is after you've exercised and cooled down. Warm muscles have greater range of motion and can therefore move and stretch easier and safely. Stretching not only allows your muscle tissues to lengthen, it also helps prevent injuries. And here's another reason to make stretching part of your regimen: healthy and flexible muscle tissue can significantly increase your ability to maintain your balance during pregnancy.

What Are The Benefits of Exercising During Pregnancy?

The benefits are endless! There hasn't been a mom-to-be who's stayed active that hasn't experienced <u>more energy, greater physical comfort, and improved psychological wellness due to exercise.</u> So, not only will it help you stay fit and healthy but it'll also help you feel beautiful and full of life.

Here are some of the benefits of exercising during pregnancy:

- **Increased Energy** – Surprising, but true. Pregnancy can eat away your energy, but exercise feeds power back into your body. It does so by strengthening your heart and other muscles. When your cardiovascular system is kept physically powerful through exercise, you can stay energized for longer periods of time.

  When your muscles are in shape, they require less energy to perform simple tasks such as carrying the groceries, walking around the neighborhood, and supporting the new life that's growing inside you. In other words, exercise allows you to preserve more energy to use and go about your day.

- **More Rest and Better Sleep** - As your belly grows, you'll discover that finding a comfortable position for sleeping becomes more difficult and getting the rest you need may seem nearly impossible at times. However, with regular exercise you'll notice that your quality of sleep improves. That's because when you are more physically active throughout the day, you are more likely to relax at night and fall asleep faster, providing you with more and better rest.

- **Decreased Pregnancy Aches and Pains** - Since exercise makes muscles stronger, it helps your body get in better shape to bear your pregnancy weight and diminish pregnancy discomfort related to muscle pain. In addition, by stretching after every workout you'll promote muscle flexibility and muscles elongation which decreases back, hip and leg discomfort.

- **Easier Labor** - Just as a marathon requires training, so do the 'long-distance' demands of labor. Giving birth requires strength, endurance, focus and commitment (coincidentally the very same requirements of this program.) Exercise delivers all these benefits. Therefore, exercising while pregnant can help you get strong and ready in order to have an easier labor and faster delivery.

- **Amped-Up 'Hormones of Happiness'** - Exercise regulates serotonin and endorphins, the hormones of happiness. By working out regularly, you'll be able to decrease and cope better with pregnancy mood swings, anxiety and worries. Pregnancy is a very touching time for a woman and exercise has proven to help all moms-to-be handle emotional demands more effectively.

- **Improved Self-Esteem** – Even though people around you are likely to comment on how beautiful and 'glowing' you are during your pregnancy, it can still be hard to maintain your self-esteem when the scale is going up, your body is growing in unusual ways, and your clothes don't fit anymore. But if you're exercising, boosting endorphins, getting better rest and not gaining excess amounts of weight, then you'll be able to focus on what's important: your health and your baby's health. When you take the time to take care of yourself and know you're doing what's right for your baby, you'll feel awesome about yourself during the nine months of gestation.

- **Recover Your Pre-Pregnancy Body Fast** - When you've kept a strong and toned body during pregnancy, you'll have an easier time bouncing back after giving birth. Your muscles will be prepared to get back to their original shape and your metabolism will be faster, which means you will be able to burn more fat for fuel. And if you simultaneously work on eating nutritiously during this period, not only will your baby be healthier, but you will too! Not to mention that you'll be avoiding the excess weight gain, cellulite and stretch marks that women who don't take care of themselves experience during pregnancy.

What Type of Exercise Can I Do While Pregnant?

Before answering this question, let me put my broken record on the turntable again: you should always consult with your healthcare provider before starting an exercise plan. Physical exertion can be taxing on the body, so you should get a 'clean bill of health' to ensure that it will not be TOO taxing for you and your baby.

That being said, if you're enjoying a low risk or normal pregnancy then **physical activity is not only safe...it's good for you!** Although you should never forget that pregnancy is not the time to get in shape or lose weight, it is however, the time to stay in the best shape possible. So, attempt to **stay physically active at least 30 minutes each day.** (This is recommended for health even when you're NOT pregnant, by the way)

My rule of thumb is this:

- If you exercised regularly before getting pregnant, then you may <u>continue your program and modify as needed.</u>

- If you weren't physically active prior to getting pregnant, begin slowly and start building up as your pregnancy progresses.

Along with the **Pregnancy Weight Workout™** you'll find outlined in the following pages, you can give your body the workout it needs by getting your blood flowing and mood elevated with:

Activities that You Can Do and Enjoy
Walking
Swimming
Resistance Training
Cardiovascular Exercise
Prenatal Yoga
Prenatal Pilates
Dancing

Listen To Your Body

Your body is an amazing thing. In addition to everything else it can do, it is very skilled at letting you know how hard and for how long you should exercise. So one of the keys for safety and effectiveness during your prenatal workouts is to learn how to 'listen' to what your body is saying and then respond appropriately.

During the nine months that you're carrying your baby, there will be some days when you feel like you could conquer the world and other days when just getting out of bed is a struggle. Why? Well, for one thing, your body is going through a tremendous number of physical changes. So as your uterus grows, for examples, it will begin to press on your lungs. This pressure makes breathing more difficult which in turn makes you get tired more easily.

On the other hand, you'll find that on certain days your increased hormone levels give you so much energy that you can clean the house, prepare the nursery, go shopping, and still have the 'zip' to put an elegant dinner on the table.

Because of this natural ebb and flow of energy that you'll experience during your pregnancy, I've broken down the workout into "Full of Energy Today" and "Not so Energized Today" sections to help you through those days.

Just listen to your body. That way you can take advantage of the days when you're feeling energized, but take it easy on the days that you're not.

Core Temperature

It's important to maintain a healthy core temperature during pregnancy, during workout time and non-workout time alike.

Core temperature, also called core body temperature, is the operating temperature deep within the body – in organs such as the liver, for example. Core temperature is different than the temperature of the tissues closer to the skin.

The normal core body temperature of a healthy, resting adult human being is 98.6 degrees Fahrenheit. Regulating core temperature is important to ensure that essential enzymatic reactions can occur. If your core level gets too high (hyperthermia) or too low (hypothermia) for more than a brief period of time, it can have a seriously negative impact on your health.

The American College of Obstetricians and Gynecologists (ACOG) recommends **keeping your core temperature below 102.2 Fahrenheit during pregnancy**. For that reason, you should

- Exercise indoors with air conditioning when the weather is hot
- Exercise outdoors before 10:00 a.m. and after 3:00 p.m., as these are off-peak hours for sun and heat.
- Exercise in a pool – swimming and water aerobics are great

The cool water of a pool is great for your body, but the elevated water temperature of a hot tub – usually set at 104 Fahrenheit – is a different story.   It may be tempting to try to soak away some of the muscle aches and pains that may accompany your pregnancy, but don't give in to temptation. Your core temperature could quickly rise to an unsafe level.

What Physical Activities Should I Avoid During Pregnancy?

Being active is important and so is being safe. Because your center of gravity changes as your pregnancy develops (due to the growing belly), you are likely to have some trouble with your balance. Therefore, it's better-safe-than-sorry to avoid activities that put your body at risk for a fall such as:

- Bicycling

- Volleyball

- Basketball

- Soccer

- Tennis

- Horseback Riding

- High Impact Aerobics

- Jogging (If you were a runner before you got pregnant, then you should be able to continue your program with caution and some minor modifications...after obtaining medical clearance, of course.

Movements to Avoid

As you learned in the Good Sense Safety Tips section, it is wise avoid lying on your back after the first trimester. That's when your baby's weight begins to interfere with proper blood flow through your arteries and lying on your back could potentially harm the two of you.

So in addition to avoiding balance-dependent activities when you're pregnant, you should also stay away from activities that include the following movements:

Movements to Avoid
Bouncing
Discordant
Jumping
Rapid Directional Changes
Abdominal Crunches

Even with all these movements and activities to avoid, there are plenty of things you can do to stay active and healthy. Let's start with one of the most important exercises there is...

Pelvic Floor Muscles & Kegel Exercises

Your pelvic floor muscles are muscles in your body that support the uterus, bladder and bowel. When they become weakened – by age, excess weight, childbirth, and pregnancy -- your pelvic organs may descend and bulge into your vagina — a condition known as pelvic organ prolapse.

Fortunately, Kegel exercises can help delay or even prevent pelvic organ prolapse and keep you comfortable. And strong, 'in shape' pelvic floor muscles will also

- **Help you carry the extra pounds** gained during pregnancy.
- **Help you during labor** by making the 'pushing' process more effective when you experience contractions.
- **Help you gain muscular control** which will help you to better relax pelvic area during labor.
- **Help you avoid the urinary leaking** and incontinence related to pregnancy.

Additionally, these movements help strengthen your pelvic floor helping you support the baby's weight with less discomfort and get your stomach back in shape after giving birth. And Kegel exercises may also be helpful for women who have persistent problems reaching orgasm.

Can you see when I'm so pro-Kegel?

The Kegel Workout

It's hard to exercise a muscle you're not familiar with, so the first thing most women need to do is discover what and where their pelvic floor muscles are. The best way to do that is to practice stopping the urination process.

The muscles that allow you to control your flow of urine are your pelvic floor muscles! Therefore in order to strengthen these muscles you need to squeeze **as if you were stopping the flow of urine, hold and then release**.

A Kegel Workout is done in four steps

- Inhale to prepare
- Exhale as you tighten pelvic floor muscles (as if you were stopping your urine flow)
- Hold as you let all the air out of lungs

- <u>Inhale</u> as you slowly release and relax muscles completely.

Aim for at least three sets of 10 repetitions a day. You might make a practice of fitting in a set every time you do a routine task, such as checking email, commuting to work, preparing meals or watching TV.

You can do Kegel exercises discreetly just about any time, whether you're driving in your car, sitting at your desk or relaxing on the couch. The time you invest in this workout will pay off handsomely before, during, and after your time in the delivery room.

The Pregnancy Weight Workout™

Okay. Now that you've learned some prenatal fitness basics, it's time to get to the heart of the matter – my just-for-you **Pregnancy Weight Workout ™**.

As you already know, the American College of Obstetricians and Gynecologists (ACOG) states that it's safe to engage in 30 minutes or more of moderate intensity exercise during pregnancy every day. That's great news! It means that in the time it takes to watch a sitcom, you can do what is necessary to stay in the best shape possible and prepare to get your body back after birth.

With an understanding that your vim and vigor will have its ups and downs during the months before you give birth I've broken down the workout in two categories:

1. Full of Energy Today: For the days in which you're feeling full of energy
2. Not So Energized Today: For the days in which you're feeling tired.

Remember; always get medical clearance before starting an exercise program. Once you have the ok and are ready to get going.

Rule #1 – Don't overdo it! Take it slowly, one step at a time, increasingly your workout time gradually. Remember, even if you start with 5 minutes a day, it won't be long before you're doing 30 minutes...or longer!

Consistency and commitment are key

Pregnancy Weight Workout

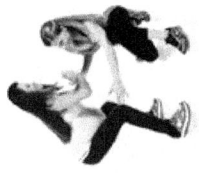

EXERCISE	SETS	REPS	DESCRIPTION
	1-3	10-15	**SQUATS** Feet shoulder width apart (dumbbells optional). Bend knees to perform squats keeping spine straight and knees aligned with heels.
	1-3	10-15	**LUNGES** Take a big step forward and distribute body weight evenly between both legs. Lift back heel and bend knees to perform lunges. Maintain front knee aligned with heel.
	1-3	10-15	**BICEP CURLS** Feet shoulder width apart holding dumbbells. Bend elbows upward to perform bicep curls. Keep back straight and shoulders engaged.

Pregnancy Weight Workout

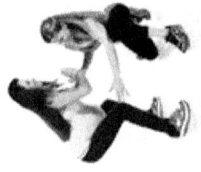

EXERCISE	SETS	REPS	DESCRIPTION
	1-3	10-15	**SQUATS** Feet shoulder width apart (dumbbells optional). Bend knees to perform squats keeping spine straight and knees aligned with heels.
	1-3	10-15	**LUNGES** Take a big step forward and distribute body weight evenly between both legs. Lift back heel and bend knees to perform lunges. Maintain front knee aligned with heel.
	1-3	10-15	**BICEP CURLS** Feet shoulder width apart holding dumbbells. Bend elbows upward to perform bicep curls. Keep back straight and shoulders engaged.

Aʙᴏᴜᴛ Fᴏᴏᴅ

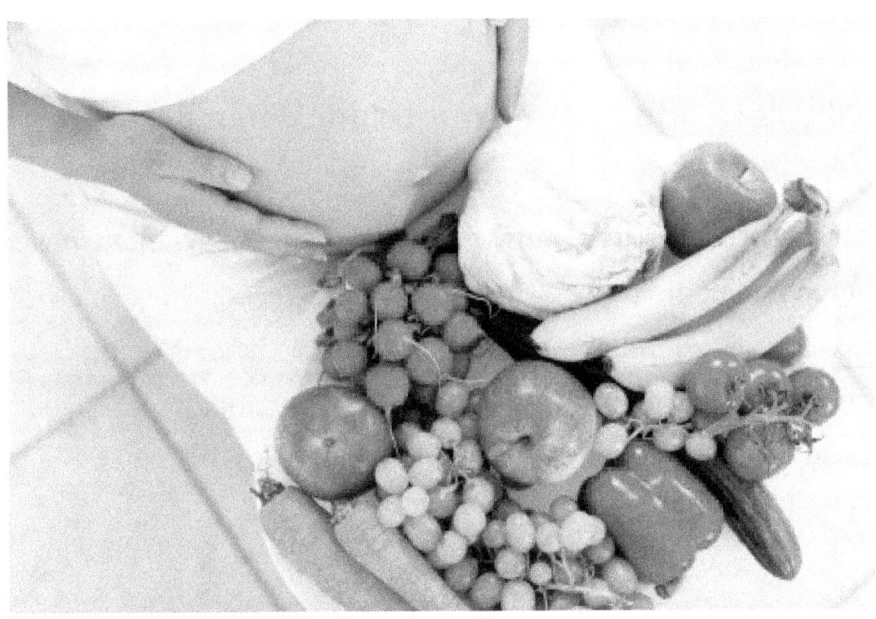

Pregnancy is <u>not the time to start a weight-loss program</u>. And on the flip side, it's not a time to throw your scale out the window and enjoy an eating frenzy that will add unnecessary excess weight to your frame. What pregnancy *is* the time to do is to **eat right.**

For your sake and for your baby's, now is the time to focus on eating appropriate proportions of the healthiest, most nutritious foods possible. This section will show you how.

About Food is devoted to your nutritional health. In the next few pages, you'll learn what to eat more of, what to eat less of, what to avoid all together and much, much more.

So please... dig in, eat up, and enjoy!

Why Is Healthy Eating Important When I'm Pregnant?

This may seem like a rather basic question, but I want to make sure you understand how truly important it is enjoy a nutritionally sound and balanced diet at this time. You are, quite literally **eating for two now**. In the incubator that is your body, your baby is counting on for all the nutrients necessary to grow and develop.

But your baby isn't the only one who needs to be well-nourished. It's been shown that conditions such as anemia and preeclampsia are more common among pregnant women who don't maintain a balanced diet.   As it prepares to bring to life into the world, your body is going through a tremendous number of physical changes and it needs a diet rich in vitamins, minerals, and other healthy nutrients to keep it strong.

In addition, there are many benefits that only a well-nourished mom and baby can experience:

- Easier Pregnancy
- Improved fetus development
- Less constipation, morning sickness and fatigue
- More energy
- Less mood swings
- Better Labor
- Faster Recovery after Labor

How Many Calories Do I Need Daily?

As I said, you're eating for two now, but that doesn't mean that you need twice the number of calories that you normally do. In fact, **your body only needs 300 extra calories per day** in order to sustain a healthy pregnancy and nurture your little one initially.

Expecting twins or triplets? Increase your calorie intake by approximately 300 calories per child.

Now once your pregnancy progresses, it's true that your metabolism will get faster. You may find that the 300 calories that were once sufficient to maintain your health and strength are no longer be enough to satisfy your needs. In other words, as your pregnancy evolves you may feel hungry more often than you did before.

Again...you need to listen to your body. If you're feeling hungry all the time or notice that your energy is low, you may have to increase your caloric intake slightly in order to satisfy hunger. That's okay! Just don't go overboard with extra calories and make sure that the calories you do consumer are from high-quality, nutritious foods...not a pint of Rocky Road ice cream.

Calorie-Counting Done for You

The grocery stores are filled with 100-calorie snack packs these days, but eating three bags of 100-calorie Oreo cookies isn't the right way to add extra calories to your diet. The sugar and fat are 'empty' calories with practically no nutrition whatsoever. (More about that in just a moment)

Instead of choosing high-calorie snacks, I recommend that you try adding a healthy, delicious extra 300-calorie *meal* to your day. The difference is that a 'meal' is a well-balanced group of foods that include protein, carbs, and fat.
A light meal can be satisfying and delicious. Here are some ideas to help you get started:

- **300 Calorie Mid-Morning Breakfasts** (be like Winne-the-Pooh and eat these for your 'Elevenses'):

- o 1 scrambled egg with 2 slice of whole grain bread and a little butter spread

- o 1 cup oatmeal, 1 cup of fruit, 1 banana

- **300 Calorie Late Lunches** (try one of these around 3:00 p.m. when the human body tends to crave 'a little something')

  - o 1 small whole grain bagel with a tablespoon of low-fat cream cheese and an orange

  - o 1 cup of tomato soup, small tossed salad with 2 tablespoons reduced fat oil and vinegar dressing, 4 saltine crackers

- **300 Calorie 'TV Dinners'** (instead of popcorn or chips, have a second dinner while watching TV)

  - o 3 ounces of grilled chicken with 1/2 cup of brown rice and steamed veggies

  - o 1 medium baked potato, 2 tablespoons sour cream, 2 tablespoons salsa, 1 cup sliced melon

Need more inspiration? Here's a website that shows just how delicious 300 calories can be: www.AdrianaMartin.com

All Calories Are NOT Created Equal

Every meal and snack you eat is an opportunity to nourish your baby with calories. But there are two kinds of calories in the world. And at this time of your life, it is vitally important that you are as conscious as you can of the difference between these two.

'Quality' calories are nutritious calories that will help your baby grow and develop while keeping you in the best shape possible. They deliver vitamins, minerals, and other nutrients in a way that doesn't spike your blood sugar or weigh you down. On the other hand, 'empty' calories are nutritionally void and useless to your body...and therefore not helpful to your baby's development.

When you eat empty calories, they satisfy your tastebuds' craving for salt or fat or sweet, but they don't satisfy it for long. Empty calories have a negative effect on your blood sugar and leave you craving more which can lead to unhealthy overeating and weight gain.

Here's a quick look at quality vs. empty calorie foods:

Quality Calories	Empty Calories
Fruits	Candy, Chips and Sodas
Raw or Steamed Vegetables	Fried Vegetables
Whole Grain Products	White Flour Products

Here's something that trips up a lot of people who are trying to eat right: sometimes the things we think of as "healthy snacks" are as healthy as we believe. The way a food has been processed can add extra calories and delete nutrients. For example:

High Calories Not so healthy	Better Option
Pastas, Crackers, Breads, Rice	Sweet Potatoes, Wheat Pasta, Brown Rice
Fatty cuts of meat such as Spare Ribs and Dark Meat Chicken	Lean Cuts of Meat, Chicken, Fish and Turkey
Fruit Juices and Fruit Smoothies	Fruit in its natural form

In my opinion, the easiest thing to do is <u>eat fresh fruits and veggies</u> for the most part and generally choose low-calorie food over high-calorie food. And if you decide to indulge your taste for something that's not super-healthy, just be sure to enjoy your treat in moderation.

Eat 'Real' Food from Mother Nature's Pantry

When I talk about 'real food,' what I mean is natural food that has been <u>minimally processed </u>instead of the food that goes through a ton of steps in order to become a product that will be sold on the shelves of a supermarket.   In a nutshell:

If you can't gather it, hunt for it, or fish for it...
it is not a NATURAL food!

The problem with processed foods is that the much of the nutritional value is lost during the manufacturing process. So the more natural and less processed foods you eat, the more nutrition you get.

You don't have to go totally 'raw' in your diet, but do

- **Consume fresh fruits on a daily basis**

- **Add more raw, as well as cooked veggies to your diet**. (Raw veggies are the most nutritious and very satisfying, too)

- **Choose fruits and vegetables that are in-season** when possible (In-season fruits and veggies arrive from local farms, losing less of their nutritional value during transit)

What Can I Do If I Only Crave Junk Food?

If you don't enjoy the taste of something then chances are you won't eat it...especially when you're expecting and your tastebuds seem to have a mind of their own. The good news is that there are plenty of delicious alternatives to the snack foods you like the most.

Healthy Alternatives for Snacking
Air popped Pop Corn (instead of chips)
Fruit: Whole, Sliced, Salad (instead of fruit pies)
Yogurt: Frozen, with Granola or Fruit, Plain (instead of ice cream)
Vegetables: Celery Sticks, Baby Carrots etc (instead of pretzels)
Nuts: Walnuts, Almonds, Peanuts etc (instead of cashews or macadamia nuts)
Seeds: Sunflower, Pumpkin

(instead of M&Ms)
Organic Almond or Sunflower Butter
(instead of processed peanut butter)

What Foods Should I Avoid?

Eating well balanced meals is important at all times, but it is even more essential when you are pregnant. There are essential nutrients, vitamins, and minerals that your developing baby needs. And while most foods are safe, there are some foods that you should avoid during pregnancy.

Let's talk about them...

High-Sugar Foods

Foods that are high in sugar contain less nutrients and higher calories than others. Since your goal is to eat 300 nutritious extra calories during pregnancy, sugary snacks and foods are not your best choice. You'll end up putting on weight, but not nourishing your body or your babies.

Here are other reasons you'll want to avoid over-doing sugar in your diet:

- Sugar during pregnancy could result in <u>gestational diabetes</u> which according to the ADA affects about 4% of expecting mothers.

- Another condition related to high sugar consumptions is preeclampsia which affects all organs of the body.

- Excess sugar consumption may cause a baby to grow excessively large which in turn increases the risk for a c-section

4 Things You Can Do to Keep a Rein on Your Sugar Consumption

- **Eat Fruit When You Want Something Sweet** – Unlike processed foods that are nutritionally empty, fruit supplies a great source of fiber and vitamins. Fruit also contains natural sugars which are digested and used by the body differently than processed sugars. Make sure to consume fruit in their natural form instead of as juices or smoothies. Fruit juice and smoothies have a high concentration of sugar, with none of the fiber of whole fruit.

- **Nip Cravings in the Bud with H20** – Did you know that dehydration may cause sweet cravings? Stay hydrated to avoid this problem.

- **Become a Mixologist -** Instead of buying sugary drinks at the store, create your own delish beverages. You can mix water with a touch of fruit juice, make herbal iced tea, add lemon, lime, or mint to a glass of water. All these beverages are wonderful and healthy substitutes for high-sugar soda or fruit juices...and healthier for your body that chemically enhanced diet drinks.

- **Know When to Say When** – When it comes to sweets, try to follow the adage that 'less is more.' It's fine to satisfy a craving for chocolate with a square or two of Ghiradelli or Nestles, just don't eat the whole bar.

Caffeine

It's been said that if caffeine were discovered today, it would be classified as a drug. It's no secret that caffeine a stimulant and raises your blood pressure and heart rate. What's less well known, however, is that caffeine is a diuretic too which causes reduction in body fluid and dehydration.

These two reasons alone should be enough to motivate you to say no to caffeine, or at least decrease your caffeine intake during pregnancy.

Coffee is not the only place that caffeine can be found. Here is a list of products that contain caffeine and should be consumed in moderation during pregnancy:

Caffeine Products
Tea
Soda, Diet and Regular
Chocolate
Some Migraine and Headache Medication

Caffeine additives are believed to make pain relievers 40% more effective in treating headaches, but the risk they present during pregnancy far outweigh the therapeutic effect.

4 Things You Can Do to Cut Back on Caffeine

- **Drink Herbal Tea** – there are so many wonderful fruity, minty, and spice-y flavors to choose from, you'll never get bored

- **Drink Green Tea** – although it has a small amount of caffeine, this antioxidant-rich beverage is much better for your than coffee

- **Drink Decaffeinated Tea and Coffee** – don't go overboard, however. Most decaffeinated products still have some caffeine in them and if you drink too many cups, you'll end up with negative side effects

- **Drink Caffeine-Free Coffee Substitutes** - Teeccino is the number one coffee alternative sold in the United States)

Alcohol

When it comes to alcohol during pregnancy just one drink may be one too many! Although, some experts say that a glass of wine every so often during pregnancy is ok, there are many of us who know that

ALCOHOL DURING PREGNANCY HAS
NOT BEEN ESTABLISHED SAFE!

There's a reason that thousands of restaurants and bars have posted signs warning women about the dangers of drinking when pregnant. Alcohol can

- Trigger premature delivery
- Cause birth defects
- Cause a miscarriage.

Furthermore, alcohol passes through the bloodstream into the placenta and on to your baby. Once absorbed, it can <u>damage the brain cells and limit the flow of oxygen to developing</u> tissues. So whenever you feel tempted to enjoy beer, a wine cooler, or another alcoholic beverage, remember this:

When *you're* having a drink, your baby is too.

Then treat yourself to a nice glass of ice water with a slice of lemon. Remember, you don't have to abstain forever. And what are a few months of going alcohol-free when it means a healthy baby!

What Foods Should I Eat While Pregnant?

If you want to increase your chances of having a beautiful healthy baby while enjoying a pregnancy and avoiding excess weight gain, eating well is your best weapon. And knowing what you *should* eat just as important as knowing what you need to avoid.

Many of the things we eat are known as '**super-foods.**' These are fresh fruits and vegetables that pack a nutritional wallop, along with their great taste and good looks. Eat plentifully from the tasty, colorful super-food 'buffet' of choices, and you and your baby will be the better for it.

Protein Super-Foods

Protein is made of amino acids that serve as the <u>building blocks of your body's cells.</u> So, it's not surprising that your baby also needs them in order to develop properly.

Do you best to <u>eat protein in every meal and snack</u> consumed through the day. And it's super important to get <u>the right amounts and the best quality protein possible</u>. What should you eat? I recommend:

Best Proteins
Chicken
Turkey
Eggs
Soy
Quinoa

Carbohydrate Super-Foods

You and your baby need <u>carbohydrates for energy and overall health</u>. But, before you load up your plate with sandwich bread, pasta, and other comforting carbs, you need to know that there are <u>types of carbohydrates</u> and the differences between them are HUGE!

- **Simple Carbohydrates** – Simple carbohydrates include staples of the American diet such as pasta, bread, white rice, pancakes, cakes etc. These processed carbs contain simple sugars have little to no nutritional value. Simple carbohydrates are absorbed quickly by the body and unless you work them off with exercise, they will just as quickly be stored by the body as fat.

- **Complex Carbohydrates** – The low-carb diet craze exemplified by the Atkins Diet made the mistake of throwing out the nutritional 'baby' with the bath water. Complex carbs -- such as vegetables, beans, whole grain products, beans -- are high in nutritional value, extremely satisfying when you're hungry, and good for you and your baby. Your body processes complex carbs differently from their simple cousins, more effectively turning carb calories into energy rather than fat.

Along with protein, you should try to eat complex carbohydrates at every meal. They will give you the energy you need to stay healthy without the excess weight gain is unhealthy. Complex carbs you can feel good about include:

Complex Carbs
Sweet Potato
Oatmeal
Whole Grain Products
Brown Rice
Couscous
Quinoa
Cream of Rice and Wheat
Barley
Yams

Fiber Super-Foods

Fiber is a key component in the digestive process during pregnancy. A woman with a fiber-rich diet during pregnancy is **less likely to suffer from constipation and other types of intestinal disorders**.

But there's another reason to love fiber. Fiber-rich foods are more filling than low fiber ones. Eating these help you feel more satisfied and stay less hungry for longer periods of time.

Fiber can be found in many foods...all of them delicious!

Fiber Foods
Broccoli
Asparagus
Mushrooms
Spinach, Romaine Lettuce and all Greens
Peppers
Whole Grains

Fat Super-Foods

Despite what you may believe, not all fats are bad. In fact, some fats are good for you and should definitely be included in your diet! Fats are satisfying and take a long time to digest. And just as importantly, they help move food through your digestive system.

Fats you can feel good about include:

Good Fats
Olive, Canola, Flax Seed and Peanut Oil
Avocado
Nuts and Nut Butters
Oily Fish (see note below)

The best fats are Omega 3's, specifically Omega 3s and Omega 6s, found in fish oily fish such as salmon. These fats are specifically important during pregnancy because they assist in the development of your baby's eyes and brain. These good fats also assist in the growth of the placenta and other important tissues.

> **Health Note**: Some types of fish contain levels of mercury which is harmful to the baby such as: tilefish, king mackerel, swordfish, fresh tuna, golden snapper, bass, bluefish and shark. Never eat raw fish while pregnant.

Calcium Super-Foods

Calcium consumption during pregnancy is essential. It helps construct and preserve strong bones and teeth in both you and your baby. But that doesn't mean that you need to down a gallon of milk every day.

Dairy calcium is good for you, but the best way to ensure that you have meet your calcium needs is by ingesting plenty of calcium-rich foods such as:

Calcium-rich Foods
Broccoli
Collard Greens
Kale
Salmon
Sardines

Vitamin C Super-Foods

Vitamin C is crucial for you and your baby during pregnancy. It helps in <u>tissue repair, injury healing, bone growth, fights infection, and other metabolic procedures</u>.

In addition to protein and complex carbs, try to consume some Vitamin C at every meal. It's easier than you think, because you can get your RDA in sweet, delicious fruits including:

Vitamin C Super Foods
Fruits: Orange, Grapefruit, Strawberry, Papaya, Cantaloupe, Mango, Raspberry, kiwi, Pineapple, Watermelon

Health Note: Your body cannot store Vitamin C, so taking a mega-vitamin supplement is not a helpful solution. Any unused Vitamin C will just pass out of your body in urine, so be sure your body gets a fresh supply of the critical nutrient daily, several times throughout the day.

What Foods Should I Stay Away From?

Some foods simply aren't good for you when you're pregnant. Let's talk about the biggest culprits:

Sugar

Foods that are high in sugar contain less nutrients and higher calories than others. Since women should eat 300 extra calories during pregnancy then its not smart to ingest them in sugary products. Moreover, too much sugar during pregnancy could result in gestational diabetes which according to the ADA affects about 4% of expecting mothers. Another condition related to high sugar consumptions is preeclampsia which affects all organs of the body. In addition excess sugar consumption may cause a baby to grow excessively large which in turn increases the risk for a c-section

Below are some great tips for cutting sugar:

- Eat more fruit. They supply a great source of fiber and vitamins besides containing natural sugars. Make sure to consume them in their natural form instead of in as juices or smoothies.

- Drink a lot of water. Dehydration may cause sweet cravings so drink up!

- Create your own delish drinks. Mix water with a touch of fruit juice or mint and substitute for soda or fruit juices

- Just a little is better than a lot. When ingesting sweet foods limit your portions that'll satisfy your taste buds but will limit your sugar consumption.

Caffeine

It's not a secret! We all know that caffeine is a stimulant and raises your blood pressure and heart rate. But, what you may not know is that it is a diuretic too which causes reduction in body fluid and dehydration. These two reasons are just enough to say no to (or at least decrease) caffeine intake during pregnancy.

Remember, caffeine is not just in coffee. Here is a list of products that contain caffeine and should be consumed in moderation during pregnancy:

Caffeine Products
Tea
Soda
Chocolate
Some Migraine and Headache Medication

Alcohol

When it comes to alcohol during pregnancy just one drink may be one too many! Although, some experts say that a glass of wine every so often during pregnancy is ok, there are many of us who know that ALCOHOL DURING PREGNANCY HAS NOT BEEN ESTABLISHED SAFE! Alcohol passes through the bloodstream into the placenta on to the baby. So, when a pregnant woman is having a drink, her baby is too.

How Often Should I Eat?

When you're pregnant, you should try to eat every 3 to 4 hours, a total of 5-6 meals a day. Sounds like fun doesn't it? Well, unfortunately, that's not always the case. I've been pregnant TWICE, myself, and I know how hard it can be to eat that frequently when you're feeling heart-burned or nauseous.

On the other hand, you may be starving from all the extra activity your body is doing in order to build a baby and eating often is easy as pie. If that's the case, your challenge is to keep your frequent meals modest and nutritious.

Whether you're struggling to eat as often as you should or struggling to keep a rein on your raging appetite, here are some tips to make your life easier.

- **If you're not feeling up for a full-fledged meal**, have a small snack instead. The last thing you want is your body having to work on fumes thought this process.

- **If you're so hungry that you can't stop eating**: choose the best quality of calories for your meals…think nutrition FIRST!

Can I Skip Meals to Avoid Excess Weight Gain?
Let me spell this out for you: N-O. Skipping meals is never an appropriate way to control weight, *especially* when you're pregnant. As a mom-to-be, you have to start visualizing that what's inside your belly is already a person. Would you let your baby cry of hunger and choose not to feed her after is born? If your answer is 'Of course not!" then you shouldn't do it while he/she is still in your uterus.

When you skip meals, you're hurting yourself...and *you* are the environment in which your baby is trying to grow and thrive. And remember, just because *you* may not feel hungry that doesn't mean your baby doesn't need to be fed. And here's something else to keep in mind...

Hurt your body = Hurt your baby =
Hurt your body = Hurt your baby...

When you skip meals, you set up a vicious cycle within your body. If you're not eating enough to keep you *and* your baby 'fed,' Nature allows your baby to take all the nutrients he/she needs at your expense, draining your reserves. This in turn creates a 'hostile environment' for your baby.

Regardless of your appetite, I urge you to keep sight of the fact that you are the only one that can take care of your unborn child at this point. It is your responsibility to do A GREAT JOB and part of that job is providing nutritional support to your child by eating regularly and eating well.

Can Food Help my Morning Sickness?

Although it's known as 'morning sickness,' many women experience "all day sickness," suffering from nausea, vomiting, or unpleasant acid indigestion at almost any hour. 75% of women go through it…so if you don't, consider yourself a lucky girl!

Morning sickness is natural and normal, even if it's not fun. Researches show that nausea and vomiting during pregnancy might be linked to:

- High level of HCG (pregnancy hormone)
- Elevated levels of Estrogen
- Stretching of the Uterine Muscles
- Digestion Ineffectiveness
- High Levels of Acid in the Stomach
- Sensitivity to Smell
- Stress

So, can eating help at all? Yes! Although food might be the last thing on your mind when you're feeling sick to your stomach, **ingesting the right nutrients can actually help minimize morning sickness symptoms.**

6 Things You Can Do to Keep Morning Sickness at Bay

- **Stay Hydrated by Drinking** - Drinking plenty of liquids can help you feel better through the day. Vomiting forces you to lose a lot of fluid which could eventually dehydrate you.

- **Stay Hydrated by Eating** - Sometimes fluids can make you nauseous and trigger a vomit response. If you're having trouble keeping down liquids, try to eat fruits and veggies with high water content such as celery, citrus, lettuce, apples, etc.

- **Eat Lots of Simple Protein and Complex Carbs** – Protein (like white meat chicken) and carbs (such as whole grain pasta) are soothing on the stomach

- **Eat Frequently** – Unless there's food to digest, the acids in your stomach will rub against its own inside layers causing you to get even more nauseous

- **Keep Your Blood Sugar Levels Steady** - Low blood sugar levels might cause nausea. Therefore it's important that you eat small meals through the day so that you can maintain these levels balanced.

- **Put Ginger to Work (Be a Spice Girl!)** – Ginger has long been celebrated for its ability to settle the stomach. Its anti-nausea properties have proven to be very successful in pregnant women. Try ginger ale, mixing real ginger in your food, and soft ginger candy chews.

Can Food Help My Heartburn?

As you end the first trimester of your pregnancy, your body will begin to produce higher levels of progesterone. This is a good thing. The progesterone levels during pregnancy is crucial for the fetus's survival, correct levels will help <u>prevent uterus</u>

contraction and blood vessel growth is promoted to give nourishment to the developing baby during pregnancy.

BUT...

High levels of progesterone also relax the muscle that separates the esophagus from the stomach. This relaxation allows the gastric acids that control digestion to filter back up. The result is HEARTBURN

You can't have a successful hormone without elevated progesterone levels, but you can minimize some of discomfort and side effects that it triggers with some simple diet changes like these...

Foods and Beverages to Avoid
To keep heartburn at bay, you should avoid

- Carbonated Drinks

- Alcohol

- Caffeine

- Chocolate

- Citrus fruits and juices

- Spicy foods

- Ingesting big meals close to bed time

Lifestyle Adjustments

These simple changes can change your pregnancy experience for the better:

- **Snuff Out Your Cigarette** - Smoking is proven to be very hard on your stomach...not to mention other parts of the body. This is a great time to kick the habit

- **Avoid Cigarette Smoke** – even a whiff of burning tobacco is enough to trigger nausea and heartburn

- **Chew Gum for Dessert** - Chewing gum stimulates salivary glands and saliva assists in neutralizing acid. Make it a habit to chew gum after eating.

- **Eat Smaller Meals** - Because your digestive process is not as efficient during pregnancy, try ingesting smaller and lighter meals that are easier to digest every three to four hours.

- **Elevate Your Body While You Sleep** - Sleeping with several pillows under your back will help elevate your torso therefore helping keep the stomach acids where they belong. (This is what people who suffer from acid reflex do.)

Why is Drinking Water So Important?

The human body is up to 60% water. The brain is composed of 70% water, the lungs are nearly 90% water, and about 83% of our blood is water.

Water is of major importance to *all* living things. And drinking enough water is crucial during pregnancy. From your increased blood volume to the amniotic fluid, water is fundamental to your health and your child's. It helps carry nutrients to your cells, facilitates the digestive process, assists in removing toxins from your body and allows your body to regulate its core temperature.

When you're pregnant, you should try to **drink half your body weight in ounces of water**. And <u>as your weight increases, so should your water intake</u>.   Pure water is the best way to go, but herbal teas and sugar-free flavored waters will also do the trick.

Just be sure to stay away from beverages like coffee and colas (including diet colas) that act as diuretics, leaching more water out of your system than they put in.

Beyond water, it's good to hydrate your body with high water foods like these:

High Water Foods
Lettuce – 95% water by weight
Watermelon – 92%
Broccoli – 91%
Carrots – 87%
Beets – 75%
Oranges – 87%
Apples – 84%
Potatoes – 79%
Bananas – 74%

What Are The Risks of Not Drinking Enough Water?

During pregnancy you should consume at least 10 to 12 glasses of water. One of the biggest reasons to stay hydrated is to avoid dehydration. Dehydration is bad for anyone, but when you're pregnant, it is particular dangerous because it can lead to:

- **Overheating** which has been related to birth defects.
- **Decreased amount of amniotic fluid** which has been related to birth defects.
- **Decreased blood volume** which prevents nutrients from passing to cells.

- **Constipation** which increases chances of hemorrhoid issues.
- **Excessive water retention** which has been linked to preeclampsia.
- **Headaches and migraines**
- **Fatigue**
- **Dizziness**
- **Cramps**
- **Premature contractions**

Now that you have a better understanding of what your body needs (and doesn't) when you're pregnant, you'll be able to use the meal planner on the following pages to ensure that maximum nutrition, along with maximum enjoyment, is the goal of every bite you take.

MEAL SUGGESTION GUIDE

Meal	Monday	Tuesday	Wednesday	Thursday	Friday	Saturday	Sunday
Breakfast	**Oatmeal pancake** Egg whites 1 serving of protein powder ½ oats Cinnamon & 1 tsp baking powder •Water	**Protein & Oatmeal Shake!** Mix protein powder oats and water in blender.	**• Protein Parfait** non-fat yogurt, 1 serving juice, ½ cup go lean cereal, Blueberries, almonds, cinnamon. • Water	•High fiber cereal •Rice or almond milk •Water	**Protein & Oatmeal shake!** •Water	•**Egg White Omelet w/ mixed veggies.** •Ezekiel Bread toast •Water	•**Natural PB&J Sandwich:** slices of Ezekiel bread •Natural Peanut butter spread •Fresh strawberries inside sandwich •Water
Snack	**Protein & Oatmeal Shake!**	**Oatmeal pancake** • Water	**Fruit Salad:** Mixed fruits with freshly squeezed lemon juice • Water	•Small apple with natural peanut butter •Water	**Oatmeal pancake** • Water	**Fruit Salad:** • Water	**Protein & Oatmeal Shake!**

64

	Day 1	Day 2	Day 3	Day 4	Day 5	Day 6	Day 7
Lunch	• Brown Rice •Black beans •Grilled Vegetables •Water	• **Sweet Baked Potato** •**Grilled Turkey** •**Vegetables** •Water	• Brown Rice •Grilled tofu strips •Green salad •Water	•Baked Potato • Grilled Tilapia •Corn on the cob Water	• 100% Whole Wheat Pasta • Tomato Sauce •Water	• **Quinoa** •Split Peas •Steamed Broccoli •Salad •Water	• Couscous • Grilled Chicken strips • Corn on the cob •Water
Snack:	•Medium size apple •Natural peanut butter •Water	**Protein Parfait** • Water	**Whole Wheat Pita Pockets** **With almond butter and organic jelly** Water	**Protein Parfait**	**Fruit Salad** • Water	Whole Wheat Pita Pockets With almond butter and organic jelly •Water	**Fruit Salad** • Water
Dinner	• 100% Whole Wheat Pasta • Tomato Sauce Water	• **Quinoa** •Split Peas •Steamed Broccoli •Salad •Water	• Couscous • Grilled Chicken strips • Corn on the cob •Water	• Brown Rice •Black beans •Grilled Vegetables •Water	• **Sweet Baked Potato** •**Grilled Turkey** •**Vegetables** •Water	•Natural PB&J Sandwich • Water	Protein & Oatmeal Shake!

This is a meal suggestion guide and should not be taken for medical counseling.

Always consult your doctor before starting a fitness or health program.

www.AdrianaMartin.com

A B O U T   Y O U !

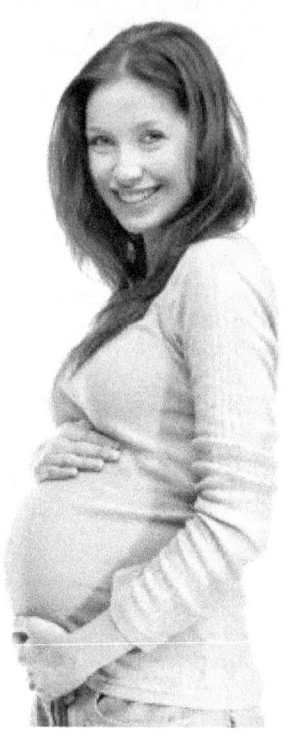

Pregnancy is one of the most amazing yet uncertain times of a woman's life. That's why it's called EXPECTING! And as thrilling as months of anticipation may be, they are also highly stressful. So in this, the About YOU section, I want to offer you a plan for taking care of yourself emotionally, as well as physically during your pregnancy.

Why Am I Feeling so Moody? Shouldn't I Feel Happy?

Feeling a little temperamental during pregnancy is normal. Think about it...your body, metabolism and hormone levels are **changing almost every day.**

- During pregnancy, your body will experience significant **changes in your hormone levels which affect brain chemicals that regulate mood**, especially during the first trimester.

- As your pregnancy progresses, more physical changes occur causing **lack of sleep, fatigue and discomfort.**

- Finally, as your due date gets closer you may began to **worry** about having everything ready for baby's arrival, being a good mom and even financial changes.

The key is being able to understand that all of these feelings are normal and that like you, there are many moms out there. You are not alone!

8 Things You Can Do to Elevate Your Mood

Knowing that other women are struggling is one thing. Knowing the things they do to feel better is another. Here are a few things that you can do in order to better cope with the tsunami of emotions that are washing over you:

1. **Saw Some Wood** – No, not literally. I mean <u>get some sleep</u>! Allow yourself time to rest and don't feel guilty for it. Your body is working overtime and it needs to be able to rest.

2. **Give Your Lungs a Workout** - As your belly grows bigger, your lungs will have less room to breathe causing you to have more difficulty inhaling and exhaling. This is counterproductive when trying to relax and manage stress. Therefore, you should make a conscious effort to <u>practice at least 10 deep breaths every time you're feeling anxious or overwhelmed.</u>

3. **Exercise to Take Advantage of Your Body's 'Medicine Chest'** - Working out helps <u>regulate serotonin and endorphin levels</u> which are chemicals related to happiness. Therefore you should always follow the **Pregnancy Weight Program**™ workout...after getting the okay from your doctor, of course!

4. **Put One Foot in Front of the other** - Walking not only promotes physical activity but it also helps take your

mind off of problems. Allow yourself some time to <u>walk outside,</u> enjoy the scenery and connect with your environment.

5. **Feel the Love** - Having the support of loved ones during this process is invaluable, but not always possible. If your mom lives in another state, if your hubby is serving overseas, or if the people around you don't understand what you're going through...then <u>join a local mother's group or chat room.</u>

6. **Give Yourself Permission to 'Screw Up'** - As women, we have the tendency to be too hard on ourselves. So if you're feeling blue, don't compound the bad feelings by beating yourself up for not having better coping skills. There are more stressed-out moms-to-be out there than you think...they just don't talk about it! <u>Allow your negative feelings to come out</u>, acknowledge them, and then and then <u>do something to turn them into positive ones</u>.

7. **Take Some 'Me' Time** - Sometimes you need to quiet your mind. When you start to feel overwhelmed, consider taking a <u>prenatal yoga class</u>, going for a <u>massage</u> or simply enjoy a cup of tea and a good book.

Little activities can help take your mind off the stresses of being pregnant.

8. **Ask a Pro** - Family and friends provide invaluable love and support, but sometimes it's necessary to get professional help, especially if what you're feeling is more of a depression than a sad, anxious or stressful feeling. If your gut is saying "Get professional advice"...do it!

What Should I Do? I Feel Anxious About My Body Changing

If dieting was part of your lifestyle before pregnancy then chances are you'll stress over gaining weight for the next nine months. Although, you know that weight gain is important to sustain a healthy normal pregnancy, you still might have a hard time seeing the number go up on the scale at every doctor's visit.

Don't worry, that's pretty normal! And here is what you can do about it:

- **Have an 'Attitude of Gratitude"** - Be grateful. Carrying, delivering and bringing a child to life is a true miracle that unfortunately many women don't get to experience. Be grateful for this moment and enjoy the process.

- **Remember that Pounds Are Only Numbers** - If you're eating healthy and staying active, then you should be gaining the proper amount of weight; Trust in the natural (and glorious) process of giving birth. Be confident that you're body is doing what it takes in order to sustain a healthy pregnancy.

- **Dress to Impress (Yourself and Others)** - Nowadays there are endless numbers of things you can do to look and feel pretty during pregnancy. Maternity clothes have never been cuter...or sexier. To give yourself a lift, you can accessorize your wardrobe with cute jewelry, mix and match your tank tops, buy scarf, hats, and shawls that 'fit' regardless of your size. Treat yourself to a manicure-pedicure.

But most of all...

- **Discover the Beauty in Your Pregnant Body** - All we truly have certainty over is the present moment, so learn to love your growing pregnant body because you don't know if you'll ever have it again.

And don't feel guilty for being focused on your weight. A major concern for many pregnant women -- and the reason you yourself undoubtedly decided to read this guide – is weight gain. While simple vanity may be the source of the concern, weight gain is an important issue to think about because of the list of potential problems that can be avoided if you keep your weight in check:

Excess Weight Problems
Backache
Gestational Diabetes
Fatigue
Leg Pain
Swelling from Fluid Retention
High Blood Pressure
Risk for C-Section
Varicose Veins

This leads to the next question...

How Much Weight Should I Gain During Pregnancy?

Good question! The guidelines vary depending on whether you were at your ideal weight, under-weight or overweight when you became pregnant. Let's break it down further:

- **If your pre-pregnancy weight was ideal** then your weight gain should be between 25 to 35 pounds.

- **If your pre-pregnancy weight was under the ideal** then your weight gain should be between 28 to 40 pounds

- **If your pre-pregnancy weight was over the ideal** then your weight gain should be between 15 to 25 pounds

- **If you're having twins** and your pre-pregnancy then your weight gain should be between 37 to 54 pounds.

Appropriate weight gain is key to a healthy pregnancy. So take advantage of the knowledge and expertise of your healthcare provider and discuss this topic with him/her.

How is the Additional Weight Distributed During Pregnancy?

While it may feel as though all the weight you are carrying is in your breasts and tummy, this graph will help you understand how your weight gain is really distributed. (The graph assumes a woman whose pre-pregnancy weight is in the 'ideal' range and who will gain 25 pounds)

Distribution	Weight
Baby	7-8 lbs
Placenta	2-3 lbs
Amniotic Fluid	2-3 lbs
Breast Tissue	2-3 lbs
Increased Blood Supply	4 lbs
Maternal Fat Stores (key for delivery and breastfeeding)	5-9 lbs
Uterus Increase	2-5 lbs
Total	25-35 lbs

How Much Weight Should I Gain During Each Trimester?

That's another excellent question. Below is a chart of the recommended weight that a woman should gain during each

3-month period. As in the chart above, the numbers are calculated based on a woman at an ideal pre-pregnancy weight

Trimester	Weight
First	1-4 lbs
Second	1-2 lbs per week
Third	1-2.5 lbs per week

These numbers are based on an average...but there is a world of difference between 'average' and 'normal.' Be sure to consult with your doctor so the two of you can decide what's right for *your* pregnancy.

How Can I Keep My Weight Gain on Track?

With this guide! The best way to ensure that you gain the recommended amount of weight is by following the **Pregnancy Weight Book™** food and exercise suggestions.

- **As far as food is concerned**: regardless of your hunger levels and cravings, keep sight of the fact that you only need an extra 300 quality calories a day.

- **And as far as exercise goes:** staying active with the suggested workout and or walking program will help you stay in the best shape possible.

How Long Will It Take to Get My Body Back in Shape?

A lot of women obsess about getting back in shape immediately after giving birth, while others give up on their bodies because they believe it's impossible to get your body back after having kids. The truth is that both of these ideas are wrong.

Here's the thing: it takes 9 long months for you to grow your body and your baby. So, it's rather foolish to think that you can get your pre-pregnancy body back in just a few weeks. (Yes, I know that super-model and Project Runway hostess Heidi Klum did it, that we all know that she's an alien...lol!)

So my message for the women who are optimistic about getting back their bodies and is the same as my message for the women who are pessimistic about regaining their former curves: if you have a healthy pregnancy without gaining excess weight then you can plan on getting your body back in approximately 30 weeks! Not bad, right?

And my **Weight After Pregnancy Program**™ will help you get in better shape than before you even got pregnant!

Will My Flat Stomach Return?

The honest to goodness truth is YES IT WILL, though it may seem hard to believe when you're bulging at the middle and carrying 25 extra pounds. It won't happen immediately, but it *will* happen.

I remember after the birth of my son Alex, I came home one night and fed him, put him to sleep, and then decided to take a shower. That was the first time I actually took my clothes off and thought about looking at myself in the mirror. To my surprise I looked as if I was 6 months pregnant, and I figured that this would be the 'new normal' in my life. It wasn't. My tummy flattened out over time.

So I always tell my first time moms, prepare to look as if you're on your second trimester right after giving birth! The good news is that as the days go by and especially if you're breast feeding, you will see your uterus shrink and shrink. Moreover, if you pair that with a healthy nutrition plan and **postnatal-specific exercises** you'll get your flat belly back before you know it!

Is There Anything I Can Do Now to Help Me Look Good Later?

Good thinking! Even though there is some work to do after giving birth, you can definitely <u>start working on your post pregnancy body now</u>! And you do that by

- Making sure to **exercise at least 30 minutes each day** (even if you're just going for a walk or stretching)

- Performing the **Kegel workout,**

- Eating the **best quality nutrients** possible in small portions every three hours.

When it comes to the pounds you gain you will easily loose the weight that's related to baby and pregnancy if you choose healthy, nutritious food now. However, if you over-eat, indulging in high-calorie and high-sugar foods, you'll be gaining excess fat and that kind of fat it's hard to lose.

If I Didn't Have a Flat Stomach Before, Is It Too Late Now?

It's NEVER too late to have a flat stomach. And it's not too late to start working on it right now. Be sure to do your Kegels to <u>develop strong pelvic muscles</u>!

By the time you give birth, your uterus is approximately 15 times heavier and that's not including the 'bundle of joy' it is carrying. The good news is that almost immediately after giving birth it begins <u>contracting on its own which makes it start shrinking</u>. A lot of women feel these post-delivery contractions, specially while breastfeeding and on the second or subsequent pregnancies.

For the first few weeks your uterus is working to get to its normal state and if you have a strong pelvic floor (thanks to your Kegel workout) <u>your body will speed up this process</u> regardless of where you were pre-pregnancy.

By the six week it should be close to its pre-pregnancy weight which is about 2.5 ounces. However, even after this happens you may still look pregnant! That's when exercise and eating healthy come into play.

Remember, your abdominal muscles have stretched and there is some work to do in order to get them back in shape. The key is to prepare your muscles while pregnant and then follow a **postnatal-specific meal and workout plan**. **The Weight After Pregnancy Program™** can help ensure that you'll look and feel better than before having kids. To find out more visit **www.weightafterpregnancyprogram.com**

Will I Be Able to Lose My Baby Weight, Regardless of How Much I Gain

You can *always* lose weight. 'Baby weight' is not hard to drop; the problem is the weight gained from overeating and ingesting too much junk and empty calories! If you gain excess amounts of weight during pregnancy will have **a harder time losing it**

As you learned in the About Food section, women who abuse sugar and unhealthy products have a higher risk of presenting complications such as gestational diabetes and preeclampsia. Moreover, babies of women who gain more than the recommended weight may be too large at birth increasing the risk of c-section. And finally, women who gain too much weight during pregnancy have **more difficulties recovering from labor** and also **problems positioning and handling the baby for breastfeeding.**

In other words, if you want to feel good before, during and after you give birth, the best recommendation I can give you is to <u>stay as active and healthy as possible!</u> This will make your weight gain ideal and will facilitate your ability to get your body back after giving birth.

Will I Lose Weight Automatically After Giving Birth?

If you gained the appropriate amount of weight during pregnancy then you shouldn't have a problem losing it soon after birth. The weight will continue to come off, day by day, as you release the excess fluid retention.

However, if the weight gain was over the ideal then you'll have to work harder at your postnatal meal and exercise plan to help shed the pounds away.

Here's the average time table:

Immediate Weight Loss	Amount
Baby Weight – lost immediately after delivery	7-8 lbs
Placenta Weight – lost immediately after delivery	1-2 lbs
Blood & Amniotic Fluid Weight – lost immediately after delivery	2 lbs
Total Weight loss	10-12lbs

I Want to Feel Good About Myself; Is It Okay to Lose Weight While Pregnant?

Let me spell this out for you: N-O! Although some women lose weight in their first trimester due to morning sickness (and sometimes all day sickness), you should **NEVER intentionally attempt to lose weight during pregnancy**! As I said at the very beginning of this book, your pregnancy is not the time to get in shape.

However, this is the time to <u>stay in the best shape possible.</u>

My Body Is Swollen; What Can I Do About It?

Although it's normal to get swollen during pregnancy it's also very uncomfortable. This swelling is <u>caused by the extra fluids circulating in the body</u> (water - blood). Also, as your baby grows so does your uterus, putting more pressure in your pelvis and therefore affecting the blood flow to and from your lower body which <u>slows down circulation.</u>

I wish I could tell you something different, but unfortunately, <u>the swelling usually gets worse towards the end of the pregnancy and during hot weather</u>.

Mild swelling of face, hands and feet is normal. However, make sure to **contact your doctor if you experience sudden increased swelling** since these are symptoms of preeclampsia (related to increased blood pressure and protein in the mother's urine).

10 Ways to Reduce that Swollen Feeling

- **Put your feet** up whenever possible
- **Avoid standing** for too long
- **Stay hydrated** by drinking plenty of water
- **Stretch often,** especially if you're sitting too long or are traveling long distances
- **Get in the water**. Whether you dive into a pool or bath tub, being in the water can help reduce swelling. But remember, you need to stay out of the hot tub since its temperature is above the recommendations for pregnancy.
- **Stay cool**. Avoid being in the heat for too long as this may increase swelling.
- **Use maternity stockings**. These help with your blood circulation. Ask your doctor for details.
- **Get a foot/hand massage**. Ask someone to rub your hands and feet upward towards your knees and elbows.

- **Decrease sodium intake**. Avoid salty foods as too much sodium increases chance for <u>water and fluid retention.</u>
- **Favor your left side.** When sleeping try lying on your left side, it will help your blood circulation.

What Can I Do to Prevent Stretch Marks?

Research shows that one of the few things that can actually prevent stretch marks is gaining the recommended amount of weight during pregnancy and at the slow pace in which is also recommended. If you pair that with healthful eating then your skin will more likely have the right amount of nutrients to keep your cells healthy and hydrated which may decrease the risk of getting stretch marks.

So once again <u>health and fitness might be the answers!</u>

Why Am I Tired All the Time?

If you're feeling tired all the time, don't worry! Feeling tired is one of the most common things that occurs to women when they're pregnant. Carrying a baby puts a strain on your entire body. Women feel the least amount of energy both during the first and third trimesters.

Let me explain more about why...

During the first trimester, fatigue feels more like exhaustion! And it makes sense because <u>your body works the hardest during this period:</u>

- Your body is building your baby's life support system – the placenta.
- Your hormone levels and metabolism are changing faster than you can imagine!
- Your blood sugar is lower
- Your blood supply increases making your heart work harder, causing your blood pressure to be lower.

Lots of changes right? The good news is that this fatigue usually ends by the end of the first trimester. And most women are able to enjoy their second trimester with lots of energy and zip. But then <u>fatigue makes a re-appearance around the seventh month</u>, the third trimester.

During the third trimester your body could start to lose steam again! Here's why...

- You're carrying a lot more weight than before
- You may have trouble moving, sleeping and doing your daily activities.

- The uterus is now bigger so it will start pressing against the diaphragm making breathing difficult which, in turn, causes fatigue.

If you feel like your fatigue is extreme and beyond normal, speak to your healthcare provider and have them check you for anemia (decreased red blood cells and/or hemoglobin). If you have anemia your blood is not carrying enough oxygen which makes you feel tired and in cases could be detrimental to you and the baby.

What Can I Do to Amp Up My Energy Levels?

Although almost every pregnant woman experiences a decrease in energy at some point or another, there are ways to help boost your stamina and keep you going as strong as possible until giving birth!

Stay Fit

Staying in the best shape possible is a key factor to keeping your energy levels up! To do that, you need to

- **Move and Move Some More** - Moving helps your stamina, so try parking far away instead of close to the entrance of the mall. Take the stairs in place of the elevator. Walk around the house when you're talking on the phone instead of plopping onto the sofa.

- **Do What You Love** - Engage in physical activities that you enjoy. This will stimulate your endorphins making your feel happy and energized. Also, engage in activities that let you feel energized (ballroom dancing) instead of exhausted and drained afterwards (marathon running).

- **Multitask** - Add prenatal friendly movements to your daily activities. For example, exercise while watching TV.

Rest

Getting as much rest as possible can help save up your energy! Recharge your batteries with:

- **Power Naps** – Naps aren't just for babies...they're for baby mamas, too. Try putting your head down for 10 to 15 minutes at a time. This will help preserve your energy levels. Oh and don't be self-conscious if you're in a public place...everyone will understand once you let them know you're pregnant.

- **Extended Night Sleep** - Allow your body to get around 10 hours of sleep at night. This might be hard to do on your third trimester with the increased size of belly and bathroom breaks so attempt to get as much rest as possible through the day.

- **Limited Drinking After Dark** - Stay hydrated, but <u>don't drink too much water close to </u>bedtime. Drinking late in the evening will cause you to wake up to go to the bathroom and that will interrupt your sleep.

Eat Well

It's a simple formula: quality eating (and drinking) will boost your energy. Try these easy steps:

- **Eat Little Meals on Little Plates** - Ingesting quality nutrients every 3 to 4 hours will help your sugar levels and therefore will keep you energized through the day. Why on a little plate? It's a trick! A small plate makes a small meal look bigger and more visually satisfying.

- **Load Up on Nutrients -** Make sure to take your prenatal vitamins and eat lots of fresh fruits and vegetables

- **Drink Up -** One of the first signs of dehydration is fatigue! So make sure to stay hydrated at all times.

Let Go

Don't try to control everything. It can be very draining and will leave you feeling exhausted! For many women, letting go can be the toughest challenge of all, but it's important that you do. And here are some tips to make it easier for you:

- **Fit Your Schedule to Your Needs, Not the Other Way Around** - You might have to take some work home or show up a little later to the office. Maybe take a longer lunch so you can sneak in a nap. Make all the changes necessary to ensure that you can meet your sleep, fitness, and diet needs

- **Don't Try to Do It All** – You're a pregnant woman, not a super woman. Ask a friend or family member for help around the house, with errands, meals, etc. so that you can rest more.

- **Take It One Day at a Time** - When the due date is getting closer, many moms-to-be feel like they'll never get the baby stuff ready on time! This sense of urgency makes women work harder which leaves them feeling exhausted. If you're going through that, make sure to focus on one task at a time and give yourself a realistic time frame. Trust that you'll get it done before the baby gets here. And if you don't, who cares? There'll be plenty of time later.

How Can I Get Better Sleep Each Night?

Sleeping sounds like a great idea during pregnancy, especially when you're feeling tired. But, with the growing belly, frequent urination, nausea, leg cramps, snoring etc., a good night's sleep is easier said than done.

So here are some healthy tips to help you get a better night's sleep

- **Say No to Stimulants** - Nicotine, alcohol, and caffeine are harmful to you and your baby, AND they can prevent you from getting a better night's sleep. Studies show that alcohol disrupts sleep patterns, smokers feel less rested than none smokers and caffeine keeps people up for at least 4 hours after ingesting it.

- **Drink By Day to Sleep by Night** - Drink more fluids through the day and less during the evening, especially closer to bed time to help reduce bathroom breaks in the middle of the night.

- **Exercise by Day to Sleep By Night** - Don't exercise late in the evening. Since exercise boosts your energy you may have a hard time relaxing afterwards. Therefore, attempt to workout at least three hours before bedtime.

- **Enjoy Your Evening Meal Early** - Avoid ingesting a big meal close to bed time as well as spicy foods since they can cause heartburn and indigestion. They'll prevent you from getting a good night's sleep.

- **Practice Breathing and Relaxation Techniques** - Begin by taking deep breaths and relaxing every single muscle in your body before going to bed. Setting aside 10 minutes every night to breathe and relax will help you fall asleep easier and faster.

- **Go to Sleep Lying on Your Left Side** - Lie down on your left side. Since this position allows blood and nutrients to pass better to the baby your body will work more efficiently and therefore your feel more comfortable and sleep better.

- **Let Music (and a Good Book) Lull You Off to Dreamland** – Watching an episode of a fast-paced television or potentially upsetting news broadcasts is not conducive to falling asleep. So turn off the TV, dim the lights, put on some relaxing music, and read a book. This process will help you relax and get in the mood for a good night's sleep.

What Can I Do if I'm Scared of Delivery?

Breathe! Most women feel a little anxious about delivery. There's plenty to worry about: the fear of not making it to the hospital on time, the fear of your baby not being born healthy with all ten fingers and toes, the fear of a c-section or other unanticipated medical intervention.

So, you see, it's normal to feel anxious. But whether or not you feel this way there is one thing you should remember:

Giving Birth is a Natural Process,
NOT an Emergency

Studies show that if you experience a healthy pregnancy by exercising regularly, eating healthy and maintaining emotional harmony then you will have an easier and more pleasurable delivery. And since you've begun that process by reading this book, you can start to relax and look forward with joyful anticipation not fear.

Conclusion

Congratulations! You've just finished a 'crash course' in having a healthy pregnancy. I hope you feel informed, inspired, and motivated to do what's right for you and your son- or daughter-to-be.

Pregnancy is a special miracle; whether through natural conception or with the help of medical science, it is still a miracle. And there is nothing as exciting or life-changing that you will ever experience.

With baby on the way, your mind may be going a thousand miles a minute. The emotional roller coaster has just begun. Your hormones are playing havoc on you and your relationships. This can be a stressful time, but you've taken an important step in making it a joyful, healthy time by reading this book.

In conclusion, I want to remind you of this...

Giving birth is the most natural thing in the world. And regardless of your fears, rest assured that your body knows how to be pregnant.

Listen to the cues your body is sending you. React and respond accordingly. Rely on loved ones for support. Take advantage of the knowledge of the team of healthcare professionals you've assembled. And remember that **the power of positive thinking will take you far on the pregnancy and parenting pathway.**

There's nothing I love more than a good 'Stork Story.' So I

hope you'll share your birth announcement with me and let me know how this book helped make your pregnancy better.

And if you need any further help or advice, I'd love to continue to be your coach, guide, and booster. You can contact me directly at www.AdrianaMartin.com

Best wishes and good luck,

Adriana Martin